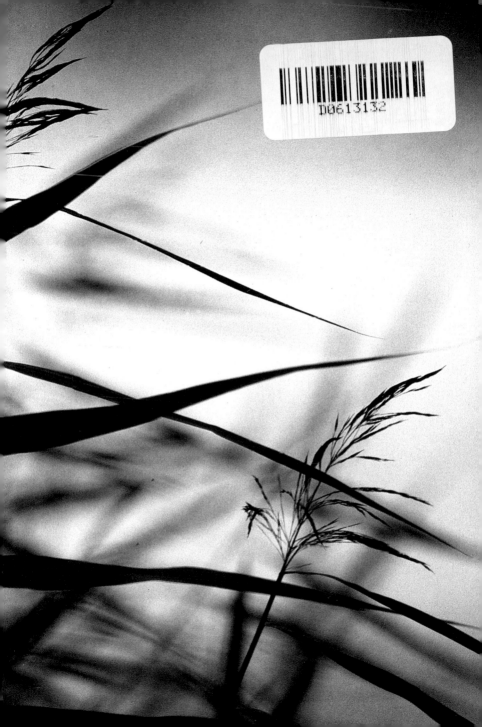

Other books by Jane Grayshon

A PATHWAY THROUGH PAIN
Kingsway 1987

A HARVEST FROM PAIN
Kingsway 1989

In Times of Pain

JANE GRAYSHON

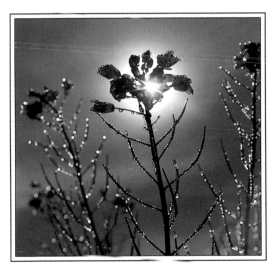

A LION BOOK

Oxford · Batavia · Sydney

Published by
Lion Publishing plc
Sandy Lane West, Littlemore, Oxford, England
ISBN 0 7459 1827 1
Lion Publishing Corporation
1705 Hubbard Avenue, Batavia, Illinois 60510, USA
ISBN 0 7459 1827 1
Albatross Books Pty Ltd
PO Box 320, Sutherland, NSW 2232, Australia
ISBN 0 7324 0194 1

Acknowledgments
Bible quotations on pages 13, 23 (third), 29 (second part), 38 are from the
Good News Bible published by The Bible Societies and Collins; on pages 17, 20,
23 (first two), 29 (first part), from The New International Version published by
Hodder and Stoughton.

Prayer on page 38 by David Jenkins, United Reformed Church's
Prayer Handbook, 1986.

Photographs by Robin Bath, pages 5, 19; Robert Harding Picture Library,
pages 25, 39; The Image Bank, page 17 /Aram Gesar, page 11 /Stockphotos
International Ltd, page 20; Lion Publishing/David Townsend, pages 31, 36;
The Photo Source/Will Curwen, Page 15; Alex Ramsey, endpapers;
David Townsend Photography, page 26; Zefa (UK) Ltd, pages 33, 43 and cover

British Library Cataloguing in Publication Data
Grayshon, Jane
    In times of pain.
    1. Man. Pain
    I. Title
    616'.0472

    ISBN 0 7459 1827 1

Library of Congress Cataloguing-in-Publication Data
Grayshon, Jane
    In times of pain/Jane Grayshon.
    p. cm.
    ISBN 0 7459 1827 1
1. Consolation. 2. Pain–Religious aspects–Christianity.
3. Suffering–Religious aspects–Christianity. I Title.
BV4905.2.G72   1990
248.8'6-dc20

Printed in Singapore

Author's Preface

'How can a *book* help someone in pain?' I wondered, when I was first asked to consider writing this book. 'I neither know each reader, nor even what their pain is! How can anyone understand what hurts someone else?' For no help is acceptable without understanding.

When I am in pain, helpful advice from others turns me off. 'They don't understand,' I groan inwardly.

Times of pain are so individual, so very personal and secret. People in pain most need understanding and personal care. Nothing I write can give that.

But then my attention was drawn to a sentence written by a child — one with special educational needs whom my mother teaches. This is what she wrote:

Pain is lonleyness becaus Know one noes what i feel

The girl was eleven. Her mother had died when she was five.

'That child has understanding,' I thought. 'She knows what she's talking about!' The writing was untidy, the letters poorly formed. Yet it seemed right. Her stumbling spelling bore the weight of authority.

I used to be a Staff Nurse in a children's ward. Those children had an astonishingly clear perspective on their suffering. Frequently, they were the ones to guide their parents towards an acceptance of their pain, sometimes even helping them to face the fact that they were dying.

Later, when I worked as a Research Sister, I listened to adults answering questions about pain. How limited they were compared with the children!

So I make no apology for quoting from children in this book. I offer some of their answers as the most expressive insights for your times of pain — whatever kind of pain that may be.

Pain is...

Pain is a horibul felling

Pain is a word for its killing me

Pain is a feeling just like gladness but pain is much sadder than gladness

Pain is the worst thing in the world

Pain is agony

My own source of pain is primarily physical. Thirteen years ago an appendix operation went disastrously wrong. I developed a severe infection which nearly cost my life, not only then but at least twice since. The infection which ensued has never been completely eradicated. Every so often things flare up, and I face pills, potions, tubes or various torments in hospital. Sometimes such episodes last for months.

The primary sympton of all this is pain. Pain has become part of my life, of my breathing. At times, when yet another infection occurs, the continual discomfort becomes almost intolerable. I feel quite unable to cope. But, as any pain sufferer knows, one simply has to. There is no way out.

Some onlookers mistake this 'coping' for bravery. Others simply say that I cannot be in pain. They have never met anyone who can 'cope' quietly. And so they dismiss the idea that I am hurting as much as they are.

Pain is so very personal. What hurts one person may barely touch another. So perhaps there is a time to accept our own pain, to hold it and maybe even hold it up to God to see what light he sheds on it. God can transform pain. But if he doesn't, he never fails to transform us.

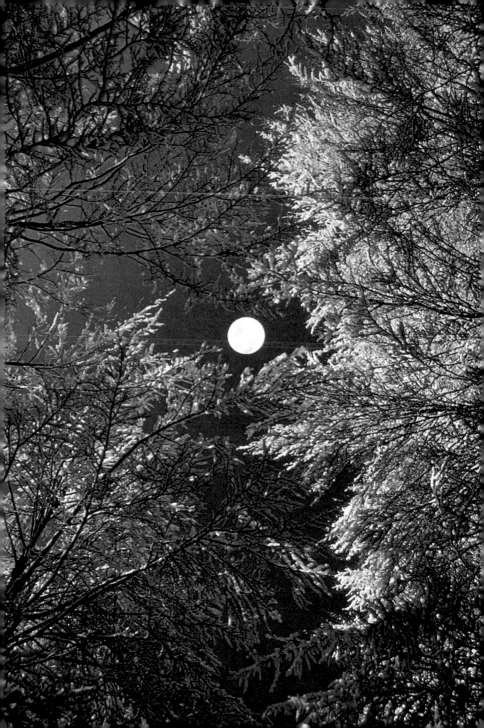

Pain's Effects

You know that your friend is in pain by the expreachion in there face

I know when my friend is in pain when he gets on my nerves

Pain not only hits where it hurts, it also invades. It causes your very self to feel under attack. It lowers resistance; it shortens tempers. Irritability is not an extra: as the children wrote so clearly, it's a part of the pain, a measure of their friend's pain.

They start to get in a bad mood

They show aggression when they are in pain

They moan a lot and mootch around the place

These children did not expect things to be any different. As one boy put it,

Pain goes all over

I wonder if, as adults, we forget this natural reaction to pain. We set ourselves an impossible ideal, expecting ourselves to overcome pain graciously and without affecting others ... then we're surprised when we do not succeed!

Newborn babies cannot explain their hunger in words. They simply cry. In moments of great anguish, we too may be unable to itemize our needs. We are as vulnerable as a baby. We need a caring parent to hear our cry and to understand what we need.

God can help pain because he is our father and he looks after us too

'Not one sparrow falls to the ground without your Father's consent. As for you, even the hairs of your head have all been counted. So do not be afraid; you are worth much more than many sparrows.'

WORDS OF JESUS, IN MATTHEW'S GOSPEL, CHAPTER 10

Trapped!

I dont know why people have pain
its impossible to guess

I dont even know why i have
pain

During my years working as a midwife, the labour
ward was a place where acute pain abounded.
    But my work was not restricted to dealing with
people in pain. There was another hallmark of this ward.
It was the place where there were births.
    In the place of most acute pain, there was also new
birth.

Not everyone sees a happy purpose to pain, even in
childbirth. Indeed, for most of us, it is the lack of purpose
in it all that hits so very hard. Pain, when it strikes, seems

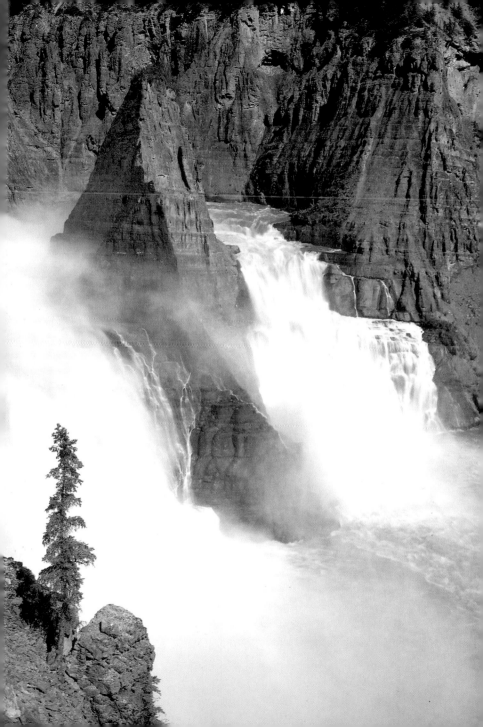

to weigh us down so much that we cannot move. We are trapped.

The women in my labour ward were trapped, too. Trapped in a clinical room, away from their cosy homes. Trapped in a bed, sometimes with their legs strapped to poles. Labour is even called a 'Confinement'.

But that did not stop the birth of new life.

Pain seems such a negative force, such a waste, it's hard to believe that anything will ever be born from it. Yet the children do not think so:

If people didn't have pain that would mean that a big feeling was missing even though it would be good to be happy all the time it wouldn't be right

I think that people need to be in pain sometimes because it is like a body function

I cannot write glibly, but I am convinced that pain accompanies birth. We may never even be aware of any fresh growth within ourselves, although we may glimpse it in others. Someone once wrote to me of a 'quiet joy' which he had watched emerge from his little boy, in pain with leukaemia. Out of pain, certain special qualities are born. Understanding, perseverance, sensitivity are

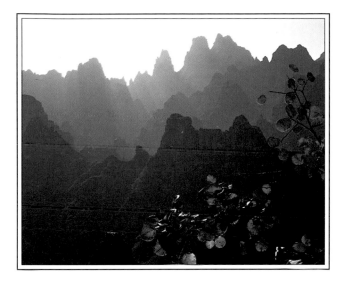

invisible — yet, like any hidden treasure, invaluable.

I suspect that all this is possible because, very often, times of pain become times when we get in touch with our own soul, perhaps as never before. They may even be times when we communicate with God himself in a new and deep way.

Jesus said: 'A woman giving birth to a child has pain because her time has come; but when her baby is born she forgets the anguish because of her joy that a child is born into the world. So with you: now is your time of grief, but I will see you again and you will rejoice, and no-one will take away your joy.'
JOHN'S GOSPEL, CHAPTER 16

How Long?

Pain goes on and on

Pain nags at you

Pain is hard to get rid of

All through labour, one of the questions which is repeated over and over again is, 'How long will it be before the baby is born?' Midwives make their clinical assessments, others speculate more randomly. Everyone is looking forward to the happy event-to-come.

Recently I was having a tooth drilled. At first the dentist was silent about what he was doing. He was taking a long time and I began to be anxious about how much more I could stand. The sound of his drill combined with the musty smell of burning until the sensation of pain

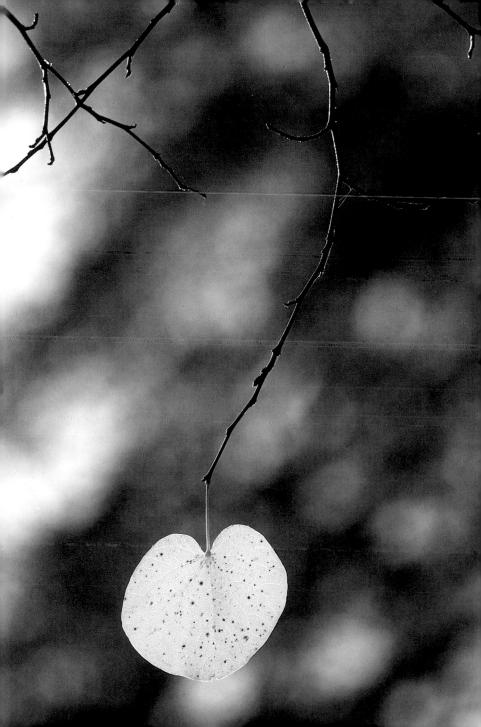

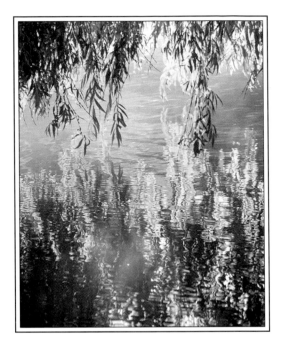

seemed much worse. Eventually I felt I could take no more
and decided I really must ask for an injection after all.
Just then, he spoke. He told me he'd nearly finished.

That simple episode was significant in my understanding of pain. It proved how easily the sense of panic
which accompanies pain can vanish completely with the
simple reassurance that it won't last for long. That is
what distinguishes times of pain from slight soreness; as
one child said:

You can't get rid of pain, but you
can have something for soreness

What is so awful in times of pain is the going on, going on with no end in sight. You don't know how you can bear it. Many people reach the stage where they feel that anything would be better than such pain.

David, who wrote many of the Psalms in the Bible, felt like that too:

'How long, O Lord? Will you forget me for ever?
How long will you hide your face from me?
How long must I wrestle with my thoughts
And every day have sorrow in my heart? ...'
FROM PSALM 13

In the absence of a time limit, simple nagging aches can turn into intense pain. During childbirth, some women reach a point where they feel unable to take any more. The question 'How long?' changes into desperation. 'I can't take any more!' This is a recognized phase, called the transitional stage.

It occurs immediately before the birth.

In God's Hands?

Campfires create a wonderfully romantic atmosphere! I recall many a time when I've grouped around glowing embers clutching hot baked potatoes and singing lustily, 'He's got the whole world in his hands...'

But has he? Does God hold our times of pain in his hands? It's one thing to sing along with friends when all is well; but pain has quite the opposite effect from romantic campfires!

Over thirteen years punctuated by times of acute pain, I have found no answer to the stark question, 'Why?' Others have given their 'answers' but none of them is watertight. Sometimes their nice answers merely serve to console themselves. Or so it seems.

The longer I continue in pain, the more my former answers are swept away.

But I have found perspectives. I do not understand what God is doing, but I do know he promises that he holds each one of us in his hands.

Hands are so different. At times they can be used against another, as when they strike a person; and it can seem that even God's hands cause us hurt at times, as if he's punishing us in some way.

Yet hands can also caress, nurture, and give expression to love. And it's this gentle and protective hold which God promises us when he says that he holds us in the palm of his hand.

'See, I have engraved you on the palms of my hands...'
ISAIAH, CHAPTER 49

Of the whole body, it is the hand which has the most nerve endings. The hand is the most sensitive part of the body. God holds us closely where he is most sensitive, feeling our every need with us.

Moreover, hands are used to guide; to assist in the creative process. One image used in the Bible is of a potter with his clay.

'We are the clay, you are the potter; we are all the work of your hand.'
ISAIAH, CHAPTER 64

To picture God as a potter, creatively moulding our lives, may help us to trust him. We may never understand all that he is doing. The prophet Isaiah expressed it like this:

'Does the clay ask the potter what he is doing?... The Lord ... says: "You have no right to question me about my children or to tell me what I ought to do! I am the one who made the earth..." '
ISAIAH, CHAPTER 45

Intense Pain

When pain has gone on longer that you can bear; when you do not know how to explain that you cannot cope with such intensity; when nothing seems to ease it, you become too drained by it to fight. You want only to die.

Some people would be better off died
Because they would not be in pain anymore

Sabina Wurmbrandt, a Rumanian Christian, was imprisoned and brutally treated for being a Jew. In prison, with other mothers, she had to tolerate hearing her children being gathered together in the cell next door to be beaten. It seemed too much to bear. 'At times,' she said soberly, 'it was just too much...'

Yet it is in those worst moments that we can stumble almost accidentally upon heaven, where it is least to be expected.

Or is it? I am beginning to wonder if this is where

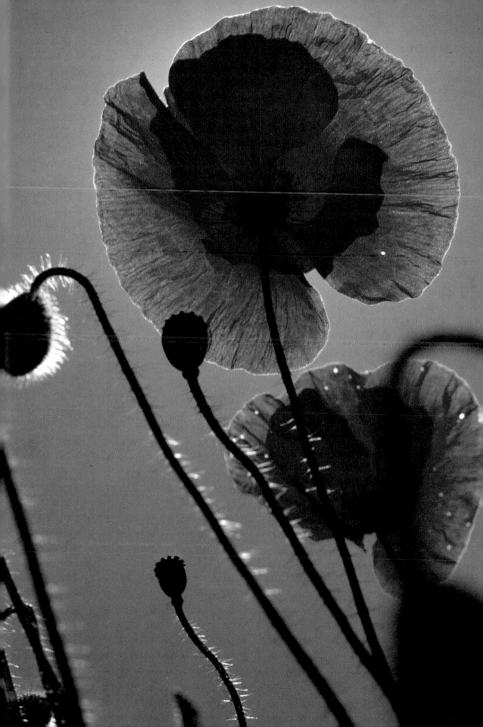

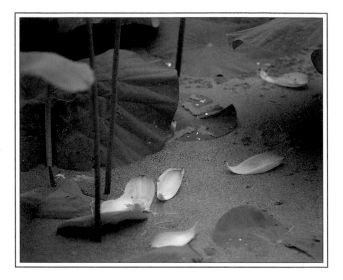

heaven is *most* to be expected... when we are past coping, where there is nothing left of ourselves — nothing left that we can do, or give, or even be.

And then God steps in.

Sabina wrote:

'At times it was just too much... But then, wonderful things happened. It seemed there was nobody there to help when at once our Lord Himself lifted away a little bit of heaven and we heard heavenly music and we saw the glory of God. When it was so hard and dark, from nowhere came this ray of light. Jesus Himself... brought light and hope and strength to forgive, and strength to go on...'[1]

[1] *Quoted from an interview with Sabina Wurmbrandt in Christian Woman, April 1988*

Not everyone experiences such colourful intervention by God. For some, his presence is much more everyday. They may not even see God's hand until, looking back, they concede that 'somehow' they have come through.

'Somehow' is possibly just a poor way to describe God's help. That we cannot say more is a reflection of the poverty of the relationship most of us have with him. We hang back from him. We may be angry that he should allow suffering; or we may be afraid to look to him. After all, intense pain makes us extraordinarily vulnerable and, for some, it is too big a risk to allow God in to where we hurt already. What if he were to make impossible demands?

But God is not like that. Jesus came, not to cast judgment on us, but to show us his love. His invitation is not for us to take a dreadful examination. He knows we'd fail! Rather, he wants us to enter a relationship with him — a relationship based on forgiveness and love.

When There's No Cure

S ome types of pain have no cure. It seems there's no hope.

Yet many children wrote of their conviction that hope does not die.

Loving and care makes my pain go better because if someone is doing that I know there is a hope

On the wall of a famous Pain Clinic in Chicago, there is a plaque which states the aim of that clinic to all who enter: 'To cure often, to relieve sometimes, to comfort always.' Or, as another child put it,

Most people take pills, but Love and care off someone close to you can take away pain

When you know you are cared-for, that knowledge alone may be sufficient to bring relief from the physical or emotional pain. But when that is in doubt, and comfort feels far away, no physical relief is felt, even when the original pain is cured.

Mother Teresa once said that the worst pain of all is knowing you are not loved. She was referring to those left destitute, whose dying bodies are ignored or kicked around on the streets of Calcutta. But we do not need to travel to India to find people who are not loved. On our very doorsteps are people whose lives are empty of love. Indeed, you may feel that you yourself bear this, the greatest pain.

Each of us longs for love and care. We yearn for comfort, if not *from* our pain, then *in* it. We long for someone to be as a midwife, to help with the pain and assist with whatever is being born.

At times, that longing runs so deep that we become aware of a thirst within our very soul. 'As the deer pants for streams of water, so my soul pants for you, O God...' (Psalm 42).

And God is not silent. He speaks to our deep need for comfort and love. He has spoken already. The comfort he offers is his presence in our pain.

'Comfort, comfort my people,
says your God...
For I am the Lord, your God...
you are precious to me and ... I love you'

FROM ISAIAH, CHAPTERS 40 AND 43

The Loneliness of Pain

Pain — especially intense pain — is very isolating. Each of us knows how easy it is to slip into a situation where pain seems to have cut us off. It's a lonely place to be.

Pain is lonleyness becaus Know one noes what i feel

In times of pain we are acutely vulnerable to the feeling that friends are letting us down. Most of us have secret hopes for help or comfort, and we feel intensely disappointed if our expectations are not fulfilled. And there's no doubt about it, family and friends do have their limitations!

Jesus knows this feeling of being let down by friends. In the worst hour of one night, he struggled until sweat trickled down his forehead like drops of blood. And his best friends slept. Three times he woke them, begging them to watch and pray. Each time they fell asleep.

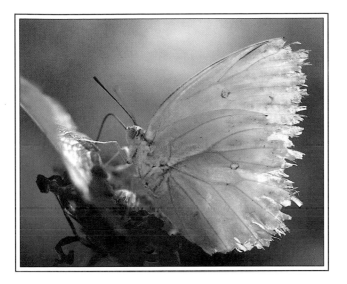

So God knows how much we need his absolute promise that he does not sleep through our times of pain. And he has given us his word. No matter how alone we may feel, we are never alone. We always have his company.

'When you pass through the waters,
    I will be with you;
and when you pass through the rivers,
    they will not sweep over you.
When you walk through the fire,
    you will not be burned;
    the flames will not set you ablaze.'

FROM ISAIAH, CHAPTER 43

Helping Others to Help

Friends and family often care, but they do not know what to do. Most obviously they want to take away the pain, so when they cannot do that, they feel useless.

If you 'cope' quietly in times of pain, they feel shut out. Their love has no channel to express itself. It's like blocking a valve, causing a build-up of pressure behind. That causes them pain. Then your friends — the very ones who should be helping you — become the ones who need help in their pain.

I believe that in the end it's you, the sufferer, who has to help them to help you. And that takes courage and understanding.

You have to be so brave that you want to make friends

Occasionally, I'm with others when my abdomen starts burning with pain. But, for some reason, I don't tell them.

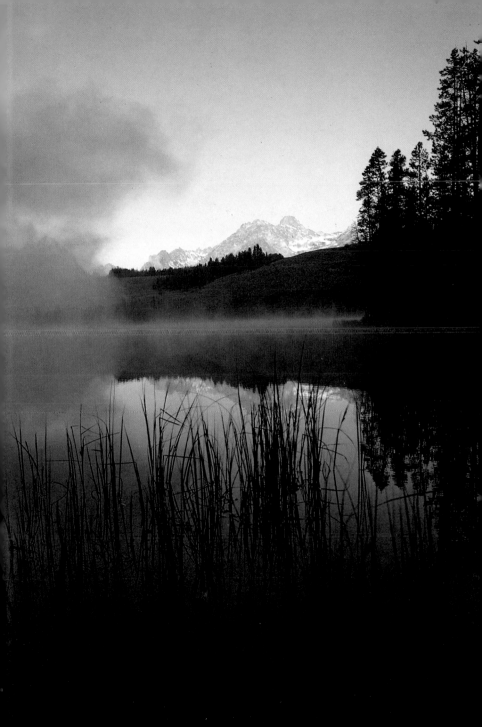

To say so, out of the blue, seems inappropriate. I wait for them to say something first. And, if they say nothing, I feel more isolated than if I had been alone. It is a vicious circle.

One child expressed this dilemma beautifully:

If you are in pain with something that you don't know what it is I think no one can help

I recall one such time when I came home, fell on my bed, and wept.

'If they had cared, they would have said something!' I cried. 'They would have noticed that I was in pain!' My tears became more bitter.

'And if they noticed and said nothing, then they really can't be concerned...'

I am beginning to see that that need not be true. Friends may notice your pain. They may care. But they may say nothing.

There are so many reasons why people say nothing in response to pain. They may be silent because you are silent. Sensitive people are afraid of 'saying the wrong thing'. They may be unsure what is 'the right thing' to say. So they hang back.

But there's more than this. They, too, may be in pain. Theirs is the pain of watching pain.

The Pain of Watching Pain

There is pain when you see someone else in pain . . . or when you watch horribal things on telivision

Others may know what you want, but be unable to give relief. They then have to bear the pain of knowing that nothing they do helps, nothing they give satisfies.

I dont think enyone can help your own pain

Friends or onlookers often say that the hardest thing for them is being unable to do anything to help a person in pain. Such impotence hurts them. They can only wait, watching.

The pain of watching may be very acute — and yet utterly private. Our families and friends themselves feel isolated. . . isolated from us in our pain; isolated in their own pain. This loneliness is hard to understand. They know all too well that they cannot fully reach another's pain.

No one can help my pain because most of my pain is in me

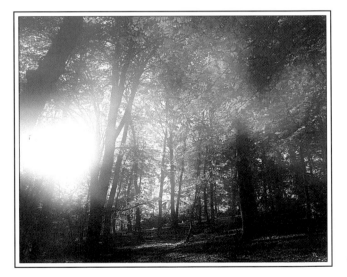

Allowing God to Help

It's not just friends who seem to get it wrong. The very existence of pain makes it look as if God has got things wrong, too.

There is spiritual pain

But it must also be true that we can either allow him to help, or prevent him from coming anywhere near us.

If God can help depends on if you believe in Him

God can help your pain. If you pray

It takes only the tiniest turning towards God for us to meet him. God does not expect us to put on a special voice to pray. He accepts us as we are: wretched, probably crying out in pain. He knows all about how we are. And he offers us all a relationship with him.

But he does not impose himself on us. God waits, watching, until we are ready to respond to him.

Jesus promised: *'I will never turn away anyone who comes to me'*.

JOHN'S GOSPEL, CHAPTER 6

Lord God,
in your compassion, come close
to those who cry out in pain,
to all who are sleepless with worry,
and to any who are physically
or mentally wounded.

Convince us that what matters in healing
is not a magic formula,
or a special form of prayer,
but simply the willingness to enlarge
our trust in your presence.

May your presence encourage
those who nurse and tend the sick
or wait and weep
as loved ones cling to life.

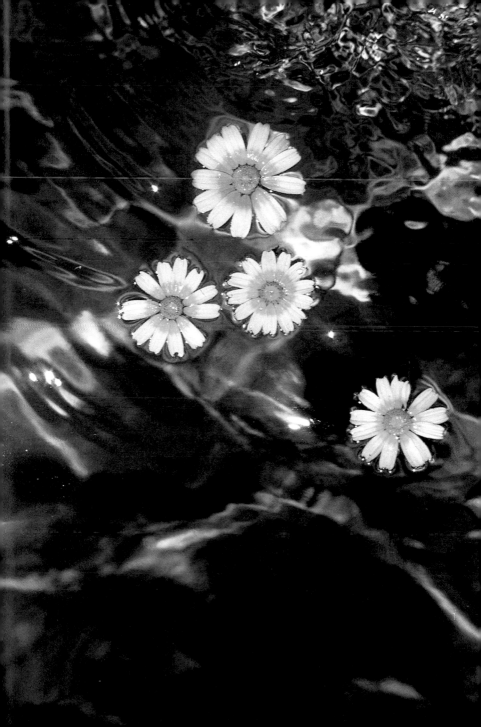

Accepting the Pain

There is a time to fight pain, when we refuse to be taken-over by it, endeavouring to overcome it as best we can. To do so requires courage which may stretch us as never before; only in times of pain do we discover inner resources which had previously lain dormant.

But I believe there is also a time to accept pain; to allow it to be built into the fabric of our being, making each of us into a more whole person.

More whole, when pain seems only to break us down? Yes, I believe so. To suffer is to be human. To be human is to suffer. Small consolation when pain seems to overwhelm! Yet pain has a mysterious dimension. It can become a platform from which we view the world quite differently. Perhaps we see it in its more rightful perspective; we begin to look at ourselves afresh; we dare to look at God anew.

This acceptance of pain cannot be forced. It may sound very grand, but it is reached through the most mundane means. Each of us knows our own little treats, our own private routines which soothe. It is when we resort to these trivial activities that we find we are taking the first steps in accepting the pain. The children's ideas of what helps them to cope are utterly practical!

Having a nice hot bath makes pain go away sometimes

My pain feels better when it's peaceful and my mum gives me a lot of attention and cares for me. And a good night's sleep as well, wrapped up in bed and the electric blanket on.

A late night helps because when my mum says you can have a late night I feel better

If you go to work and keep hard at what you are doing you forget about it

Watching television or reading a book can make you feel better

Company so I can talk to them and I will forget about my pain

If you are in pain like a head ace a pill would fix it

A doctor can help if he is a speshelesr

Few children mentioned the drugs that kill pain, except as an afterthought. I would want to endorse that philosophy, although I must stress that that is a personal decision in which the doctor must be the closest adviser. Drugs are the least of what helps. And yet, with that, I have to confess that most of this book has been written between injections of diamorphine!

Two of the children offer a remedy for pain that is starkly simple:

Company from my mum

Antybruyotics

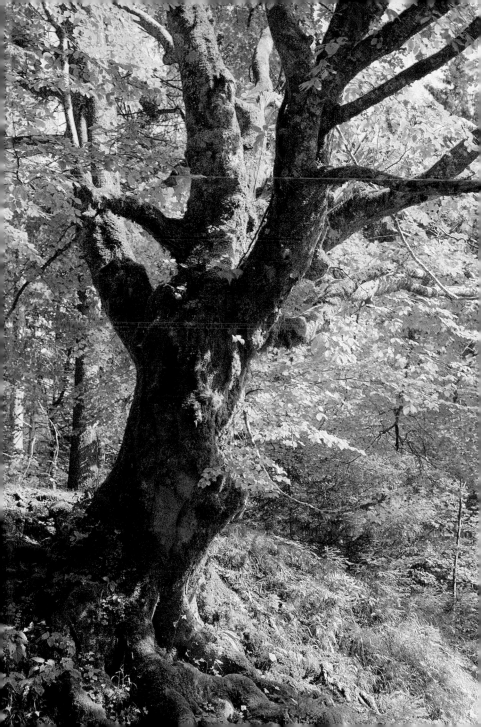

Closeness

In times of pain, you yourself are like an open wound. You can bear others to come near to you only if they are going to be soothing. As when a wound is bathed with cotton wool, you need them to be sensitive and careful. You need them to avoid causing more hurt. If you suspect that someone may brush past, may come near without the essential soothing balm, you want to keep them as far away as possible.

So you may be intensely lonely in your pain, yet you may be keeping others away lest they cause you more hurt.

For the same reason, people sometimes want to keep God away.

'If you're going to let me hurt like this, I don't want you near in case you make things worse!'

Only those who truly understand are allowed near. More often than not, they are the people who have been through intense pain themselves.

They are the ones who know that slick answers are empty. They are the ones who cannot say, 'Never mind,

dear. You'll be better soon.' They know that that may not
be true. They are the ones who wait and weep with you;
who hold you until you have the courage to look up and
wipe the tears from your eyes. It is that secure hold which
is often stronger than words. Those who truly understand
will simply stay with you, sharing your times of pain.

I have found God to be the one above all who
understands, upholds and stands with me. In times of
pain, I hold to his promises.

What God gives to me, he promises to all who turn
to him.

'I will never leave you;
I will never abandon you.'

HEBREWS, CHAPTER 13

'Don't be afraid or discouraged,
for I, the Lord your God, am with you
wherever you go.'

JOSHUA, CHAPTER 1

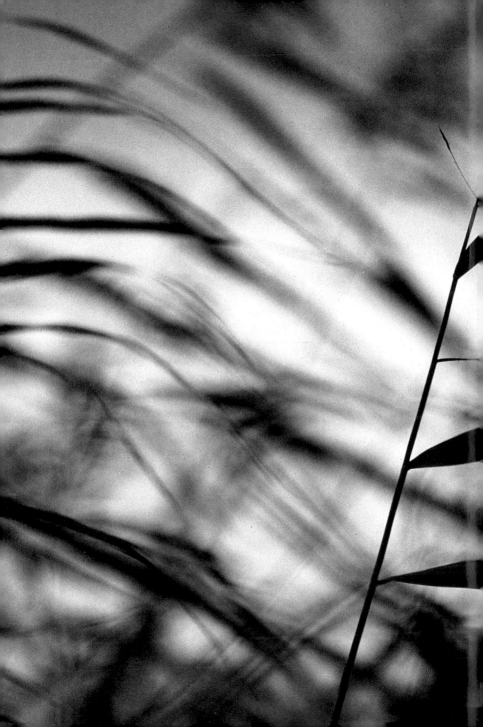